THE GREAT BIG BOOK OF BOOBS

Everything you need to know about Breast Augmentation

First Edition

By Matt Goldschmidt, MD
Independence, OH
The Cosmetic Surgery Center

JONES MEDIA PUBLISHING

The great big book of boobs: Everything you need to know about Breast Augmentation

Independence, OH The Cosmetic Surgery Center.

Jones Media Publishing
10645 N. Tatum Blvd. Ste. 200-166
Phoenix, AZ 85028
www.JonesMediaPublishing.com

ISBN: 978-1-945849-20-6 paperback
First Edition: May 2017

Contents

Acknowledgments

I am grateful to Jeremy Jones and his staff at Jones Publishing for all of their assistance with this project. I would especially like to thank Adam Kosloff for all of his contributions and editing of this book. Without his masterful help and insight, none of this would have been possible. I would also like to extend my gratitude to my close friend, Melinda Pavlik. Her input from the other side of the proverbial table, has never gone unnoticed. I am indebted to her for all of her input, thoughtful suggestions, and of course her commitment to cosmetic surgery. Likewise, her support, was invaluable to this book. I also wish to thank my wonderful parents, Paul and Janice, and my children, Abby and Marissa, who provide unending inspiration.

Introduction

The prospect of having cosmetic surgery evokes strong emotions.

You might be *excited* to remake your look, *nervous* about what the actual process will be like, *confused* about whether to go forward, or *scared* because you read something dubious on the Internet about the subject.

I wrote this book for breast implant candidates—to put your mind at ease, help you feel confident in whatever decision you make, and give you insights so that you can feel in control.

While this book isn't medical advice, I do have significant experience in this field. In addition to owning and running The Cosmetic Surgery Center in Cleveland, Ohio, I am a practicing, expert cosmetic surgeon; an examiner for the American Board of Cosmetic Surgery; and a medical lecturer and author. I have had the privilege of helping thousands of women (and men too!) feel better about their bodies, performing procedures as diverse as breast augmentations, liposuction, tummy tucks, facelifts, breast lifts, eyelid surgery, facial fillers, Botox, and many others.

The Big Book of Boobs will give you a "20,000 foot" perspective and raise and answer questions that many people have had about the process.

If you have specific questions, my team and I would love to help. Please call us at (216) 264-8100 to schedule a private consultation, or learn more about us and how we help people feel great at www.drmattgoldschmidt.com.

Enjoy the book!

What is Breast Augmentation Surgery?

BREAST AUGMENTATION, ALSO KNOWN AS "augmentation mammoplasty," is a surgery used to increase the size, shape, or fullness of the breasts. Over 400,000 breast augmentation surgeries are performed in the United States every year.

Patients choose breast augmentation surgery for many reasons. Some wish to make smaller breasts larger or to create a more symmetric appearance. Pregnancy, weight loss, and breastfeeding can dramatically alter the breasts; surgery can restore their original fullness and shape. Breast cancer, trauma caused by serious accidents, and other events that require the removal of part or all of the breasts also motivate women to get this surgery.

The Basics of the Procedure

We will explore the technical elements shortly, but here's a thumbnail sketch. The surgeon inserts breast implants under the muscles of the chest or the already existing breast tissue. These implants—made of silicone, saline, or other materials—replicate a wide range of feel, firmness, and shape. Their flexibility makes breast augmentation an option for a wide range of patients.

Some people crudely refer to breast augmentation surgery as a "boob job," but this dismissive language does a disservice to patients by downplaying the significant, lasting positive effects of the procedure.

Studies show that patients who choose breast augmentation surgery report high levels of satisfaction. For instance, a 2013 study in Plastic and Reconstructive Surgery found that 98 percent of patients surveyed said that they got the results they expected. Women also reported that they felt more confident, that they had better self-esteem, and that their overall quality of life had improved significantly following the procedure.

In addition, 85 percent of the patients surveyed thought their post-surgery size was "just right," and 99 percent were satisfied with the way their scars had healed. The study also found that most patients were back to living their normal lives less than a month after surgery.

Why Choose Breast Augmentation?

WHAT INSPIRES PEOPLE TO OPT for breast augmentation surgery? The catalog of reasons is surprisingly diverse. Let's consider a few of the most common:

1. **To restore breast size and shape after pregnancy or breastfeeding.**

According to the American Society of Plastic Surgeons, in 2013, patients ages 30 to 39 received 105,877 of the breast augmentations performed in the United States—or one of every three procedures.

Women in this age range are typically in the middle or end of their childbearing years. The hormonal and structural changes the body endures during pregnancy and breastfeeding can radically alter the size, shape, and feel of the breasts. Reduction in size and firmness is especially common. Since there are no exercises or creams that can restore fullness, many people opt for breast augmentation once they are finished having children.

2. **To correct asymmetry, genetic chest deformities, or the results of an accident or illness.**

Breast augmentation is a form of reconstructive surgery; as such, it addresses a wide range of medical problems, including:

- Dramatic breast size variance;
- Congenital deformities in chest development;
- Injuries or damage caused by accidents or illnesses;
- Aesthetically unwanted changes caused by surgery to treat conditions like breast cancer.

3. **To improve confidence and comfort.**

Conventional wisdom preaches that "beauty is found on the inside" and cautions that superficial changes to one's appearance will lead (at best) to superficial levels of satisfaction. Obviously, there is no one key to self-confidence, and complex factors contribute to our psychology, ranging from early childhood experiences to hormonal/neurological issues to diet and nutrition.

That said, the science is surprisingly clear: studies show that the overwhelming majority of patients who opt for breast implant surgery report increased self-esteem, more confidence, and a sense of being more comfortable or "at home" in their bodies after recovery. These changes in self-perception and happiness endure over time, according to analysis.

Obviously, surgery is certainly not a substitute for other techniques (e.g., therapy, medication, mindfulness practice, etc.) to address confidence and self-esteem issues. But it really shouldn't be that shocking to consider that making positive changes to your appearance can lead to positive downstream psychological effects. Our bodies and our minds are tightly intertwined.

Breast augmentation that addresses sagging or asymmetric breasts can also increase physical comfort too, and make life simpler in surprising ways. For instance, some women can now buy clothes "off the rack," without needing to pay for and wait for alterations.

A Brief History of the Field

ALTHOUGH BREAST IMPLANTS HAVE BEEN around for less than 75 years, breast augmentation surgeries have a much longer history—and not all of it is pleasant! We have come a long way.

The first breast augmentation surgery is typically dated to 1895, at the University of Heidelberg in Germany. The doctor, Vincent Czerny, was working with a patient who had just had a large benign tumor removed from one of her breasts—leaving the breast with a radically different size and shape than its partner. Discovering that the patient also had a lipoma, or large fatty deposit, in her hip, the doctor removed the lipoma from her hip and inserted it into the damaged breast to reconstruct it and restore symmetry.

Also in the 1890s, an Austrian surgeon started championing the use of injected paraffin to enlarge breast size. Unfortunately, the use of paraffin turned out to be ineffective as well as dangerous. The injected paraffin could migrate, causing a large, oddly shaped lump. It could also cause ulcers or even blindness.

In the 1920s and 1930s, experiments to create safe, stable breast implants involved materials ranging from glass balls to beeswax to Teflon. Silicone was first used widely for breast implants in the 1940s, but the silicone used was rarely sterile, as medical-grade silicon is today. When this silicone was injected with nothing to contain it, the results sometimes led to damage and infection.

The 1950s saw the emergence of implants made of polyvinyl or polyethylene. While these materials didn't lead to the catastrophic medical effects of paraffin or injected silicone, they also didn't last long. When they failed, patients often found themselves looking and feeling worse than they had before surgery.

The first silicone and saline implants were developed in the 1960s. The patient who received the first set of silicone implants, Timmie Jean Lindsey, still has them today—in her 80s. After silicone implants were recalled in 1992, saline implants became standard in the United States.

In 2006, the FDA approved silicone gel-filled implants designed to avoid the problems that got the earlier silicone implants recalled. Today, if a silicone gel implant breaks, the gel is semisolid and is contained by a shell that gives the implant its shape. It is not able to "leak" into the patient's body. Both silicone gel and saline implants today come in a wide variety of shapes and sizes, increasing the possibilities and options for patients who seek breast augmentation.

What Makes Someone a Good Candidate?

OVER 400,000 BREAST AUGMENTATION SURGERIES are performed in the United States every year. Are you a good candidate for this procedure? The following factors suggest that you might be:

- **You have realistic expectations for the procedure, informed by a qualified surgeon.** Be sure to research and evaluate alternative nonsurgical interventions.
- **You have fully-developed breasts.** Most doctors recommend against performing breast augmentation surgery on adolescent patients, whose bodies are still developing.
- **You are in good general health.** Patients fighting severe illnesses/infections or have diseases that compromise their immune system should avoid having surgeries that are not specifically intended to address their medical problems.

Patients who have untreated breast cancer should not get breast augmentation surgery, although they may be candidates for surgery after the cancer has been treated.

- **A qualified doctor has assessed your chest muscles and breasts and searched for contraindications.** Undiagnosed breast conditions can cause serious complications or require your surgery to be postponed or canceled. Abnormal mammograms should be followed with additional examination or testing as needed.
- **You are not allergic to any material used in the implants or during surgery.** Inform your doctor and surgical team of any allergies to medications or other substances. Some allergies, like a latex allergy, can be accommodated during surgery with the use of latex-free gloves and other devices.
- **You are willing to listen to and abide by your doctor's instructions regarding postoperative care.** You need to follow such guidelines to avoid risks and dreaded complications.

When Is Breast Enhancement Surgery NOT Appropriate?

BREAST AUGMENTATION MAY NOT BE the right choice for you if:

1. **You are still in your teens.**

Teenagers, especially those under the age of 18, are still growing very quickly. Since growth can affect the size, shape, fullness, and placement of the breast implants, wait to perform any augmentation until the breasts have had a chance to fully develop.

2. **You are pregnant or breastfeeding.**

Pregnancy and breastfeeding can dramatically change the breasts. Surgery during these times can be hard on the body, dangerous for a developing baby, or damaging to your ability to provide the nutrition your little one needs. Once you reach the end of pregnancy and breastfeeding, however, you may be a good candidate.

3. **You haven't had a checkup for breast health recently.**

Undiagnosed medical conditions or abnormal mammogram readings may contraindicate breast augmentation surgery, because surgery could make the condition worse. Make sure your existing breast tissue and chest structures are healthy before undergoing surgery.

4. **You have untreated breast cancer, or you are battling breast cancer.**

Breast augmentation surgery before or during breast cancer treatment could have negative effects on your health and complicate your recovery. Coordinate with your oncologist to determine the most appropriate course of action.

5. **You have a serious illness or infection.**

Illness and infection stress the body's ability to defend itself and recover from trauma. Patients with untreated medical problems put themselves at risk for unwanted complications. Further, patients with poorly controlled diseases that affect their immune system may risk poor healing or infection of the implant. Talk to your surgeon about your ailments, and then schedule an appropriate time for the procedure.

6. **You aren't informed about the limitations and requirements of breast augmentation surgery.**

If you don't know what to expect, you may be disappointed or confused by the results. Ask lots of good questions beforehand. Consider compiling a list of all your concerns and sharing them with your doctor. For future reference, write down the answers you get.

What Are the Most Common Risks and Side Effects?

LIKE ANY SURGERY, BREAST AUGMENTATION poses certain medical challenges. Patients may experience side effects from the implants or from the medications used during surgery or postoperative care, or they may experience risks during the procedure itself.

Breast Implant Risks and Side Effects

These include:

- **Rupture and deflation of saline implants.** When a saline implant ruptures, the saline is absorbed by the body, since it closely matches the body's own electrolyte balance. However, the implant will deflate as saline leaks out. Most patients then notice that the effected side does not fill out their bra like it usually does and looks smaller than the uneffected side.

- **"Silent rupture" of silicone gel-filled implants.** Today's silicone implants are a semisolid substance and are designed to not "leak" into the breast tissue or patient's body. However, a rupture can cause symptoms in some patients, including hardness of the breast and discomfort. Others may experience a "silent rupture," with which there are no symptoms.
- **Pain.** Pain may be caused by "capsular contracture," in which the scar tissue that normally forms around the implant becomes tight and begins to put pressure on the implant and breast tissue. Or pain may be caused by nerve damage or changes in the muscles. In some cases, the pain is idiopathic—it has no identifiable cause.
- **Problems with breastfeeding.** Many people can breastfeed after augmentation with no problems. But in some cases, internal scarring from implant surgery can interfere with breastfeeding.
- **Additional surgeries** to correct problems such as scar tissue or rupture. In some cases, surgery may be needed to remove or release the scar tissue and place a new implant immediately.

Breast Augmentation Surgery Risks and Side Effects

In addition to risks from the implants themselves, the surgery to insert them can pose certain risks, just as any surgery can. These include:

- **Adverse reactions to anesthesia, medications, or other substances.** It is vital to alert your doctor to any allergies you have and medications you are taking, so that the surgery team can avoid using medications that interact badly with your current medications and avoid exposing you to known allergens.
- **Scarring or problems with wound healing.** Although one study found that only 1 percent of breast augmentation patients disliked their scars, risks can occur when incisions are made.

- **Hematoma and other postsurgery complications.** A hematoma is a collection of blood near the site of the surgery. Whenever breast surgery is performed, there is a risk of hematoma, which can also cause swelling, bruising, and pain. The body may take care of a small hematoma on its own, but larger ones may need to be drained by a medical professional. It is critical to follow your doctor's instructions carefully to minimize the risk of these problems.
- **Increased risk of infection.** Although hospitals and surgical centers work hard to keep operating and recovery rooms as clean and sterile as possible, surgeries can and do increase the risks that germs will invade and an infection will result. If you have a weakened immune system, you may be at higher risk of getting an infection.

What Are the *Uncommon* Risks and Side Effects?

THE COMMON RISKS AND SIDE effects of breast augmentation include implant rupture, scarring, nerve injury, capsular contracture, and postoperative infections. However, rarer risks and complications can occur as well. Here's a short list of concerns:

- **Breast Tissue Atrophy.** In some cases, the body responds to the breast augmentation with a thinning and shrinking of the breast tissue.
- **Calcification or calcium deposits.** Hard lumps of calcium may form around the implant, under the skin. While they are not harmful, they can be uncomfortable. They might also be mistaken for precancer or cancer in a mammogram image.
- **Extrusion.** Like tissue atrophy, extrusion involves a breakdown of the breast tissue or the skin. However, an extrusion ends with

the implant poking through the place where the skin has broken down.

- **Blood clot.** Blood clots typically form in the lower extremities during surgery. These blood clots are then called "DVTs," or deep venous thrombosis. They can be life threatening if a piece of the clot were to break off and travel to the lungs (pulmonary embolus). Fortunately, this risk is extremely rare in breast implant surgery. Be sure to advise your surgeon of any significant personal or family history of bleeding problems or blood clots.
- **Lymphedema or Lymphadenopathy.** These conditions involve swelling or enlargement of the lymph nodes. Since lymph nodes exist throughout the body, the condition can affect any of them, including those in the chest or underarms.
- **Necrosis.** Necrosis is dead skin or tissue around the breast. The risk is increased by infection, use of steroids in the breast pocket, smoking, and chemotherapy or radiation.
- **Seroma.** A seroma is a collection of fluid near the site of the surgery. Like a hematoma, it can cause pain or discomfort. Intervention to drain the site may be needed if the seroma is large. Textured implants may also raise the risk of seromas.

Should you be worried? While these outcomes do happen, they are unlikely. Ask your doctor about specific concerns you have, along with his or her personal history of patients encountering these problems.

Myths about Breast Implant Surgery That Need to Be Dispelled

TYPE THE WORDS "BOOB JOB" into your favorite search engine, and you'll find useful information about breast augmentation surgeries—but you'll also find a lot of myths, half-truths, and "horror stories." To make a fully informed choice about your own surgery, you need to separate myth from fact.

Here are some popular myths about breast implants, along with the facts you need to know:

Myth: It's going to be obvious that my breasts are "fake."

Fact: Breast implants can be tailored to your body to produce a natural shape, size, and feel.

Breast implants have come a long way since they were first introduced in the 1950s. Today, careful planning with your surgeon can ensure that your breast augmentation is tailored to your height, weight, and natural breast size and shape. The most common reasons implants looks "fake" — choosing too large an implant for your body type/size or placing a saline implant in front of the muscle—can be avoided.

Myth: I'll have to have my implants replaced in 5–10 years.

Fact: Unless a problem occurs, replacement generally isn't necessary.

The recipient of the first silicone breast implants received hers in 1964, and she still has them today! Unless the implant leaks, ruptures, or causes other problems, it can stay in the body. Many people have the same implants for twenty years or more.

Myth: Breast implant surgeries cause ugly scarring.

Fact: Scarring can be kept to a minimum, and most people are not bothered by their scars.

A 2013 study in *Plastic and Reconstructive Surgery* asked 225 women to discuss their breast augmentations. Less than 1 percent of them reported feeling self-conscious or uncomfortable about their scars. In most cases, scarring can be kept to a minimum and hidden by the natural curve of the breasts. Scar treatment can also help to fade the scars faster.

Myth: My implants will fix droopy breasts.

Fact: Another type of surgery may be needed to fix "droop."

If your nipples sit at or below the bottom of your breasts, an implant alone will not raise their profile. Instead, talk to your doctor about having a breast lift surgery. A lift can be performed instead of an augmentation or in addition to an augmentation.

What Incision Options Are There?

JUST AS THERE ARE SEVERAL options for type, size, and shape of breast implants, there are also several options for where the incision will be made to insert the implants. The choice depends on a number of factors that you should discuss with your physician.

Here are the most commonly used incision options:

Inframammary: Below the Breast

Inframammary incisions are made in the fold beneath the breasts. They provide easy access for inserting nearly any type, shape, or size of implant, so your surgeon can do the best possible job in placing the implant and practicing careful surgical techniques. Scarring is often minimal, and any scars that do appear are often hidden beneath the fold of the breasts, so they cannot be seen even when you are not wearing clothes.

Periareolar: Around the Areola

This incision is made at or around the areola (the pigmented skin surrounding the nipple). While the scar is often easily hidden, especially on people with dark areolas, this incision can disrupt the milk ducts, making it harder to breastfeed. It is also not appropriate for all types or sizes of implants. This incision may also disrupt the feeling in the nipple or areola.

Transaxillary: Under the Arm

An underarm incision can be hidden well and often heals with little or no scarring. However, this form of insertion prevents the surgeon from seeing exactly where the implants are being placed. Therefore, the risk of asymmetrical results (breasts that are a different size, shape, or height from one another) is higher with a transaxillary incision.

Transumbilical: Through the Navel

Also known as a "TUBA" procedure, these types of insertion procedures are much less commonly used in breast augmentation surgeries. They can only be used with saline implants, and like a transaxillary incision, this option does not allow the surgeon to see exactly where the implant is being placed. Other options tend to produce better results. In addition, a small incision under the breast may also be needed to facilitate the surgery.

Several methods are available to help your incision heal with minimal scarring, no matter where it is located. If you have questions about the incision, potential scarring, or any other part of the procedure, don't hesitate to talk to an experienced surgeon.

Types of Implants and How to Choose the Right One

BREAST AUGMENTATION SURGERY HAS DEVELOPED significantly from its early days. Today, there are more options available than ever for finding the look and feel you want.

However, having all these options available can feel overwhelming at first. Which implants should you choose? Here is a guide:

Silicone vs. Saline: How Do They Differ?

The two most commonly used types of implants are silicone breast implants and saline breast implants. Silicone implants are filled with silicone gel, which feels similar to natural breast tissue when the implant is inserted. The FDA has approved these implants for use in patients ages 22 and older.

Older silicone implants made headlines in decades past when they ruptured, causing the liquid silicone to leak into the body. Current implants are designed to prevent this problem because they are semisolid and are also intended to trap any "escaping" silicone.

Saline implants are filled with sterile salt water. If the implant leaks, the saline is simply absorbed by the body, since it is not much different than the body's own fluids. The effected side will slowly appear smaller than the intact side. The uniform shape, firmness, and feel of saline implants still makes them popular. The FDA has approved them for use in patients ages 18 and older.

Choosing the Right Implant for You

Since silicone and saline implants vary slightly in terms of feel and shape, the one you choose will depend in part on the size and overall "look" you wish to achieve. Your doctor can help you understand which effect each type of implant will have on your look.

Because saline implants are designed to deflate if they rupture, a ruptured implant may give you a significantly "lopsided" look until it is replaced.

Silicone implants can also rupture, but they will not deflate when they do. This is known as a "silent" rupture. Follow-up appointments for MRI imaging or other tests are generally required to make sure the silicone implant is seated correctly in the body and there are no problems. Naturally, if there is a problem with silicone implants, additional surgery may also be the best option to correct the problem—but such problems are unusual. Most people enjoy the benefits of breast implants for many years without complications.

Important Vocabulary Patients Should Know

WHEN YOU EMBARK ON THE journey of undergoing breast augmentation surgery, you begin to hear words and phrases that aren't part of your usual vocabulary. Just like traveling to a foreign country, traveling to the "world" of breast augmentation is more comfortable and interesting when you understand the local language! Here are some of the top terms you should know:

Areola: The pigmented area of skin surrounding the nipple.

Augmentation mammoplasty: Another name for breast augmentation or breast implant surgery, in which the size of the breasts is enlarged or enhanced.

Breast implants: Medical devices that are placed inside the body to reconstruct the breasts or to enhance the size of existing breasts. These implants are typically made either of saline or of silicone.

Capsular contracture: A complication that occasionally occurs after surgery. Scar tissue surrounding the implant tightens, squeezing the implant. This usually results in a very hard breast that can be painful and/or disfiguring. Capsular contractures typically require further surgery to release/remove scar tissue and place a new implant immediately.

Hematoma: A collection of blood that has pooled beneath the skin around the implant. In some cases, a small hematoma may resolve on its own after surgery; in other cases, the area may need to be drained by a doctor.

Inframammary incision: A cut made under the breast in order to insert an implant.

Mammogram: An X-ray image of the breast. Mammograms are used to screen for breast cancer as well as to evaluate whether you are a good candidate for a breast augmentation surgery.

Mastectomy: A surgery in which some or all of the breast tissue is removed, from one or both breasts. This procedure is one of many responses to breast cancer, when it is used to remove diseased tissue.

MRI: An abbreviation for "Magnetic Resonance Imaging." This test is similar to an X-ray, in that it creates images of internal tissues. It is generally painless.

Periareolar incision: A cut made at the edge of the areola in order to insert breast implants.

Submammary or subglandular placement: Breast implants that are inserted directly behind the breast tissue and on top of the pectoral muscle.

Subfascial placement: Breast implants that are inserted underneath the muscle fascia (a very strong layer that surrounds the muscle). The implants are on top of the muscle but separated from the breast tissue by this tenacious tissue.

Submuscular or subpectoral placement: Breast implants that are inserted under the pectoralis major muscle, which is located behind the breast tissue.

Sutures: The stitches that hold skin and tissue together after an incision is made.

Transaxillary incision: An incision or cut made under the armpit in order to insert breast implants.

Ultrasound: An imaging test, similar to an MRI or an X-ray, that uses high-frequency sound waves to create an image of the interior of the body. This test may be requested to further characterize a spot on a mammogram to better understand the spot in question. It can help determine if further treatment is needed, such as a biopsy.

Determining the Right Size Implant

CHOOSING THE SIZE AND SHAPE of the implants you want to use in your breast augmentation surgery can be a great deal of fun. We work with you to choose the implants that will give you the size, shape, and profile you want. Here's how:

Trying on Breast Implants

One approach we take is to ask you to bring a few different tops to your appointment. Then, we have you "try on" implants by placing them in our special sizing bra. This method can help you see how the implants will fill out your bra (and your tops), and it helps your doctor narrow down the best size, shape, and materials for your implants.

Measuring Your Breast Width

At your appointment, your medical team will also measure the width of your breasts. Typically, this width is measured (in centimeters) from the inside to the outside of the breast in a straight line. Breast width is one significant consideration in choosing the right implants for your body, since the best choice is typically an implant that is the same width as your breast or slightly narrower.

Breast Tissue Considerations

The thickness of breast tissue varies from person to person. For the most natural looking and comfortable results, the size of the implant should accommodate the thickness of the tissue as well. For instance, a person with thicker tissues can often choose a wider implant better than someone with thinner breast tissues.

Can I just tell you what cup size I want?

While cup size can help provide a ballpark understanding of the general size you are looking to achieve, relying on cup size alone is not likely to get the results you want. First, the size of the bra's cups doesn't communicate any information about the shape of the breasts, how they will move, or where they will sit on your chest. All of these factors are essential to the overall "look" you wish to achieve.

Second, every bra company sizes its bras differently. What one company calls a 36DD, another might call a 34C. What matters is that the implants fit you and that when you look in the mirror, you like what you see! It is more important, once all is said and done, that you like what you see and not so much what the tag on the bra says. Depending on where you shop and buy your bras, the size will greatly vary from store to store.

How Much Does Breast Augmentation Cost?

THE POPULAR MEDIA HAS MADE breast augmentation seem like a luxury item, priced out of reach of anyone but celebrities and well-off individuals. In fact, a breast augmentation performed by an experienced and qualified surgeon is highly affordable.

According to the American Society of Plastic Surgeons, the average cost of breast augmentation surgery is about $5,800. Surveys of breast augmentation prices nationwide reveal a range of $3,600 to $8,500, depending on the type of implants used and on other factors.

Factors that influence the cost of a breast implant procedure include:

1. **Type of implants used**

The type and size of the implants can affect the cost of the procedure. Currently, most breast implants contain either saline or silicone. Your doctor will work with you to choose the size, shape, and material for the implant that will produce the effect you want. You'll know which implants will be used—and thus be able to get a sense of their cost—before the day of your surgery. Some manufacturers may have additional fees for their warranty coverage that you may be responsible to pay. Be sure to ask what your warranty covers and if any additional warranties need to be purchased.

2. **Specific steps included in the procedure**

Some breast augmentation procedures involve simply inserting implants. Others include a "lift," which affects the position of the breasts and the profile of the chest. If you are having an augmentation after a mastectomy, injury, or other event that has changed or damaged your chest area, your doctor may need to contend with scar tissue or other complications. Naturally, the more complex the procedure is, the more you can expect it to cost.

3. **Hospital and anesthesiology fees**

In addition to the costs of the implants and of working with your surgeon, there are costs related to anesthesiology, hospital care, and your visit to the operating room. Your doctor or your hospital of choice may be able to help you plan for these fees.

4. **Costs insurance doesn't cover**

Since breast augmentation surgery is frequently considered a "cosmetic" surgery, many health insurance plans do not cover it or cover only some of the expenses related to it. To avoid being surprised by the size of the bill, talk to your insurance company, so you know which costs are and are not covered.

How Should Patients Prepare for Surgery?

THE DAY FOR YOUR BREAST augmentation surgery is close at hand, and you're probably feeling a mix of excitement and nervousness. You can help the procedure go well and speed your own recovery time by taking steps to prepare for surgery.

Your doctor will likely give you specific instructions on preparing for surgery. You should put these guidelines first when you prepare. However, you can also keep general preparation guidelines in mind, including:

1. **Get a good night's sleep.**

Surgery puts stress on the body, so adopting healthy habits can help your body face the challenge. Get plenty of sleep before your procedure. Also, clear your schedule for several days after the procedure, so you can rest. Consider stocking up on your favorite books, movies, or other quiet activities, so you aren't tempted to overextend yourself.

2. Eat a healthy diet ...

Prepare your body for your procedure by giving it the nutrition it needs to speed healing. Focus on getting plenty of vitamins and minerals. Adding fruits and vegetables to your routine is one easy way to do this. Also, drink plenty of water to keep yourself well hydrated.

3. ... but remember to stop eating and drinking when your doctor instructs you.

As important as good nutrition and hydration are before surgery, it's also important to go into the procedure on an empty stomach. Otherwise, you may suffer complications from anesthesia. Focus on feeding your body what it needs until the point your doctor recommends that you fast, and then avoid food or water until after the procedure.

4. Stop smoking.

If you smoke, it is best to stop for at least four to six weeks before your surgery. This further reduces stress on the body and helps normalize your responses to certain medications. If you do not quit smoking until right before surgery, you may also risk complications from anesthesia.

5. Follow your doctor's instructions about taking medications.

Your doctor may ask you to stop taking certain medications, such as aspirin, nonsteroidal anti-inflammatories (ibuprofen, Aleve®, Motrin®, Advil®, etc.), and certain vitamins and supplements before your surgery. This is because some medications can change how your anesthesia works or affect bleeding and clotting. Likewise, if your doctor instructs you to take any medications before your surgery, take them on time.

If you have questions about preparing for surgery, don't hesitate to talk to your doctor. It's the best way to know what's ahead and minimize your recovery time and risk of complications.

What Implant Placement Options Are Available?

IN ADDITION TO CHOOSING THE right size, shape, and material for your implants, you and your doctor will discuss the best placement for the implants during a breast augmentation. Currently, three main options are used in breast augmentation procedures.

Subpectoral, or "Under the Muscle"

Also known as "submuscular," this placement inserts the implants beneath the pectoralis major muscle—the fan-shaped muscle that sits on the chest beneath the breast tissue. (Remember doing "we must increase our bust!" exercises during middle school slumber parties? You were exercising the pectoralis muscles.)

Because this placement puts both the muscle tissue and your breast tissue over the implant, it can hide the upper portion of the implant and make the outcome less obvious. Saline implants are often inserted under the muscle, because their shape and firmness can make them "stand out" without the added pressure of the muscle to keep them within your body's profile.

There are a few disadvantages to this placement as well. Since the surgery itself requires intrusion under the muscle, many patients report that recovery takes longer and feels more uncomfortable. Also, when the chest muscles are flexed, they can put pressure on the implant, temporarily changing its shape—an effect called "animation distortion." While the implant goes back to its regular shape when the muscle relaxes, this change can be a concern for some people, especially if they are particularly athletic. Over time, the effects of the muscle on the implant may result in pushing the implant downward and toward your armpit. This may require further treatment to surgically reposition the implant.

Subglandular or Submammary

A subglandular placement might also be called "submammary." Here, the implant is placed on top of the pectoralis muscle, but directly underneath the existing breast tissue.

Silicone implants are commonly inserted using this method, because they often do not need the added coverage of the muscle to produce a natural shape. Whether they choose silicone or saline implants, many women who already have a moderate amount of breast tissue also prefer this placement. The recovery is also shorter and less painful for many patients.

So what are the drawbacks? First, the implants can be seen and felt more easily, especially if they contain saline. Second, some "rippling" may be visible in the implants in some thinner patients.

Subfascial

When implants are placed on top of the muscle but underneath the fascia of the pectoralis muscle, we refer to this as "subfascial placement." Fascia is a thin but extremely tough layer of connective tissue that surrounds muscle bundles and other anatomic structures, to help keep them separated from adjacent tissues. Placing the implants underneath the fascia helps keep the implant from separated from the overlying breast tissue. By placing the implants subfascially, the patient has less recovery (compared to subpectoral placement) and lower risk of capsular contracture (compared to subglandular placement). This placement may also help patients who do not want the "high and tight" look that may be associated with subpectoral implants. Additionally, subfascial placement may also reduce the risk of the implants appearing far apart. The main drawback of this placement is that thin patients will exhibit more rippling or wrinkling in the upper part of the breast. Newer highly cohesive gel implants may reduce this risk and be optimal for subfascial placement.

Your doctor can help you choose where to place the implant, based on your body, the implant type, and implant size, along with the results you want to achieve.

Should Implants Be Placed Below the Muscle?

FOR MANY YEARS, MOST SURGEONS who performed breast augmentations preferred to place the implants beneath the muscle, a procedure also known as a "submuscular" or "subpectoral" placement.

This placement is still used, and for the right patient, it can be the best choice. However, it is not the only option. Depending on the type of implant, the shape and quantity of existing breast tissue, and the results you are looking for, either subpectoral, subfascial, or subglandular placement may be used.

Why Should an Implant Be Placed below the Muscle?

Reasons your surgeon might recommend placing your implants below the muscle include:

- **You have very little existing breast tissue.** Placing the implant below the muscle puts more of your own body's tissues over the implant, helping it to appear as if it is also part of your body's natural structures.
- **You're also planning to have a "lift."** A breast lift is a procedure that addresses sagging. For some patients, the best results come from using a "below the muscle" placement in addition to the lift.

The main drawback to placing the implants below the muscle is that the procedure is harder on the body, and it requires more recovery time. For you, this may mean added pain and more time spent away from activities you enjoy.

When Should I Consider Having Implants Placed Subfascially?

When saline implants were the most common type used, the below-the-muscle placement was the most common choice as well. Today, however, both the cohesive and the newer highly cohesive ("gummy bear") gel implants can be placed on top of the pectoralis muscle (subfascial) with excellent results.

An over-the-muscle placement is often a good choice if:

- **You have moderate amounts of breast tissue.** The implant can be used to blend in with your existing breast tissue, providing a natural-looking result that takes full advantage of your existing breasts.
- **You've chosen silicone gel implants.** These implants are designed to work well when placed subfascially. Your doctor can help you estimate what the results will look like.

Most patients report less pain and faster healing times with subfascial placement of their implants. However, the implants may be easier to see and feel in this position. Talk to your doctor about the right choice for your body, your lifestyle, and the look you want to achieve.

Will Your Breast and Nipple Sensitivity Change?

ONE OF THE BIGGEST QUESTIONS that comes up during discussions about breast augmentation is "How will implants change the feeling in my breasts and nipples?" While many people who consider implants do so because they want to *feel* sexier, no one gets implants so they can actually enjoy sex less.

Here's what you need to know about sensitivity and implants:

1. **You probably won't lose sensitivity—and you may even gain some.**

You should still be able to feel your breasts and nipples after a breast augmentation. Total numbness is extremely rare, if ever seen. Most patients will report that initially after surgery, they have less-than-normal feeling in their breasts/nipples. Subsequently, many report they have extrasensitive nipples, and then they usually revert back to the preoperative sensation. The majority of patients lose no breast or nipple sensitivity in the long term. Many even report that their sensitivity increases, and that being touched is *more* enjoyable once their implant incisions have healed. We will typically recommend patients take a vitamin B complex to help the nerves heal faster.

2. **Loss of feeling is often related to pressure on the nerves in the chest.**

When nipple or breast sensitivity decreases after an augmentation, it's typically due to one of two causes. First, use of an incision around the nipple can decrease nipple sensation in some patients. If this is a concern for you, talk to your doctor about alternative sites for the incision.

Second, sensitivity may decrease if the nerves are stretched extensively. This happens most often in people who opt for a significant increase in size all at once. To decrease this risk, you can choose a smaller size or plan to increase the size of your implants in stages instead of in a single procedure. Your doctor can help you plan this transition to decrease the chances of losing sensitivity.

3. **What you feel immediately after surgery isn't what you'll feel when you're fully healed.**

In the first few days and weeks after implantation, your body is adjusting to the presence of the implants and the disruption to its everyday functioning, which results from any surgery. As a result, sensations in your chest area may be entirely "out of whack." You may feel numb some days and sensitive or even "tingly" on others. Some patients may even report an occasional "electric shock feeling" that happens for a moment at random times. Your sensitivity will change as your pain and swelling decrease, and as your nerves adjust to the presence of the implants.

What Happens, Step By Step, in a Typical Procedure?

HUNDREDS OF THOUSANDS OF BREAST augmentation surgeries are performed in the U.S. each year. For most of these patients, the procedure follows a set of typical steps, with expected results and no serious complications. Here are the steps your surgeon is likely to follow in any typical procedure:

1. **Anesthesia**

First, you'll be given medication to help you be comfortable during the procedure. There are several different anesthesia options, including intravenous sedation or general anesthesia. Talk to your doctor if you have any concerns about anesthesia, as well as about which options are best for you.

2. **Incision**

Your surgeon makes an incision so that the implant can be inserted. While inframammary (under the breast) incisions are most common, other incision options are available. Talk to your doctor before you schedule surgery, so you know your choices and what to expect.

3. **Inserting and Placing the Implants**

After the incision is made, your doctor will insert each implant into a pocket created under the breast and/or muscle. Depending on the type of implant, your existing breast tissue, and the look you want, the implant will be placed either underneath the pectoral muscle (i.e., subpectoral/submuscular) or on top of the muscle but under the fascia (i.e., subfascial).

4. **Closing Incisions**

Once the implants are placed, and your doctor has checked to ensure they are well-seated and symmetrical, the incisions are closed. Sutures are used in the deeper tissue layers, and the incisions through the skin will be closed with sutures, adhesive, and/or surgical tape. Although incisions can look rough immediately after surgery, the lines fade as the skin heals over time.

5. **Postoperative Care**

Once the procedure is finished, and your incisions are safely closed, you are taken to a postoperative care area. You may be given additional medications to control nausea, pain, and other forms of discomfort as you wake up from anesthesia. Generally speaking, patients who have a breast augmentation procedure are able to go home as soon as they are awake, and it is clear that they have no major complications from the surgery.

6. **Recovery**

Your doctor will give you a list of instructions to follow as your body heals. These may include rest, use of medications or a pain pump, and guidelines on how to care for the incision sites. Some patients will receive a compression bandage to help minimize the risk of bleeding. Others may need to have a special band placed on top of the breasts to help them settle in faster. You will be given instructions that are appropriate for your specific procedure.

How Long Does Recovery Take?

ALTHOUGH GREAT STRIDES HAVE BEEN made in recent decades to make breast augmentation surgery a safer and less invasive experience, all surgeries have some recovery time.

The First Two Days

For most patients, the hardest part of the recovery period occurs in the first 48 hours. During this time, you'll want to watch closely for any signs of bleeding or other problems at the incision sites. You may start to develop bruises.

Best Practices during This Time: Take medications as directed by your doctor. Follow instructions carefully, including any advice on wearing a support or sports bra, moving your arms, or taking care of incision sites. Watch for signs of bleeding or of infection, like redness, tenderness, or fever. Cancel any plans, and get lots of rest.

The First Two Weeks

During this time, you'll be able to move around more and even take showers. You may still have fluid retention and swelling, as well as constipation from certain types of pain medication. While your pain should decrease, you might find that you still need some medication at night.

Best Practices during This Time: Limit your physical activity; always do less than you feel you can do. If your doctor has given you exercises to do, start these on schedule. Follow instructions for incision care carefully, and stay alert for any signs of bleeding or infection.

Weeks Three and Four

During the third week, your pain should continue to decrease, and your swelling should decrease with it. Most people can start doing low-impact exercises again around the fourth week, although it's still wise to avoid high-impact or resistance exercises for your upper body. You may have some unusual nerve sensations, like numbness or "pins and needles" feelings.

Best Practices during This Time: Decrease your pain medication, and start moving around again as your comfort permits. Continue to do any exercises prescribed by your doctor and to wear a support bra if you need it. If pain, swelling, numbness, or tingling cause trouble, talk to your doctor.

The First Nine Months

Although you may feel fully healed by the end of the first month, your body is still adjusting to the implants for up to nine months after surgery. Your scar tissue will relax, swelling will resolve, and your breasts will become softer. You'll also see the biggest differences in your self-image.

Will You Need to Replace Your Breast Implants?

BREAST IMPLANTS CAN IMPROVE SYMMETRY, enhance your body's shape, and provide a great confidence boost—but they are not intended to last forever. Most manufacturers recognize that saline breast implants will likely need to be replaced every 10 years. If you are fortunate, and your implants have not deflated and are without problems, then you do not necessarily need to do anything simply because you have reached the 10-year mark.

Does this mean you need to plan a new surgery every decade? Not necessarily. On the one hand, statistics for saline implants say you will likely need to replace them within 10 years. On the other, the first person to receive silicone implants had her surgery in the 1960s—and still has the same implants today!

Signs You May Need a Breast Revision

- You may need to replace your breast implants if:
- You have saline implants that have deflated,
- An X-ray, ultrasound, or MRI indicates that your silicone implants have a leak or rupture,
- You want to change your implant or breast size,
- Your implants have shifted, or the scar tissue around the implants has tightened (a condition known as "capsular contracture"), or
- Stretching, weight loss or gain, or other events have changed your breast tissue.

What to Do If You Think You Need Replacement Implants

First, talk to an experienced breast augmentation surgeon. Your doctor will order any imaging he or she believes is necessary. Ultrasounds or MRIs can help you and your doctor see the state of your current implants and make any needed plans to replace them.

Generally speaking, you are a good candidate for a replacement or revision if you are in good health, if you do not smoke, and if you want to address issues with your current breast size, shape, or the results of your original implant procedure.

Planning and preparing for an implant replacement is similar in many ways to having a breast augmentation for the first time. You'll talk to your medical team about the size, shape, and feel you want to achieve. Your doctor will review the records from your first surgery and make any needed plans to adjust or address certain problems, like scar tissue, sagging, or implants that have moved out of position. You and your doctor will discuss options like implant type, placement, and the incision to be used when replacing your implants. And, of course, you'll need to plan ahead to have the needed rest and recovery time after your procedure.

Breast Implants: Pregnancy and Nursing Challenges

MANY PEOPLE WHO CONSIDER BREAST augmentation worry about how their implants might affect their pregnancy or their ability to breastfeed a baby—or how the changes pregnancy and breastfeeding cause will affect their implants. Here's what you need to know.

Will my implants change my ability to breastfeed?

For most people, breast implants have no effect on the ability to breastfeed. Implants are inserted in the body behind the breast tissue, including the glands that produce breast milk—which means that the implants can stay as they are, without ever affecting your ability to produce breast milk for your baby. Your implants will probably not make breastfeeding any harder or easier. If this is a critical factor, it is best to avoid any/all elective breast surgery until you have finished having children and nursing. If you plan to pursue breast implant surgery prior to this, it would be best to avoid a periareolar incision ("nipple incision") to prevent injury to the milk ducts.

Concerns about silicone gel implants in the early 1990s led to a number of studies about the effects of silicone in the body, including studies that sought to find out whether the silicone could get into breast milk. According to a 1999 survey of the research, (https://www.ncbi.nlm.nih.gov/books/NBK44780/), there was little or no evidence that silicone from breast implants affected breast milk in any way. In fact, one study found that there was more silicone in some infant formula brands than in the breast milk of mothers who had implants.

Will pregnancy or breastfeeding change the shape, position, or feel of my implants?

The breasts go through a lot of changes during pregnancy. If you have implants, it's natural to wonder whether those changes will affect them.

Generally speaking, although the breasts do tend to get bigger during pregnancy, this change in size will not affect your implants. Reports of patients who found their implants painful due to pregnancy-related changes are extremely rare. In fact, many doctors have never met a single person who had this problem. Likewise, breastfeeding should not affect your implants in any way.

Remember though, that while the shape, size, and feel of your *implants* does not change during pregnancy or breastfeeding, the shape, size, or feel of your *breasts* may change. Pregnancy and breastfeeding do change the breast tissue. If these changes are significant enough, you may find that you dislike the size, profile, or feel of your breasts after pregnancy. If this happens, talk to an experienced breast augmentation surgeon about your revision options.

How to Choose the Right Breast Implant Surgeon for You

FOR YOUR PROCEDURE, YOU'LL WANT a doctor who is certified; who has experience with the type of procedure and implants that will be best for you; and who makes you feel informed, prepared, and completely comfortable. Here's how to start your search.

Finding a Surgeon

Wondering where to start looking for a surgeon? Try these resources:

- **Your family doctor.** Your family doctor, OB/GYN, or primary care physician may be able to refer you to local surgeons who focus on breast augmentation. Once you have a referral, however, don't hesitate to follow up by asking questions. Make sure the referred doctor is the right one for you.

- **Professional organizations.** Organizations like the American Society of Plastic Surgeons or the American Board of Cosmetic Surgeons keep databases of their member surgeons, and can also provide helpful tips on how to choose among your options.
- **Word of mouth.** Both online sites like RealSelf.com and connections with people in your area can help you find out whether a particular surgeon's patients were comfortable in the office, knew what to expect, and are happy with their results.

Choosing the Right Surgeon for You

Once you've narrowed down your list of options to a few promising names, it's time to start talking to potential surgeons one on one. Here are the most important questions to ask a potential surgeon:

- **What credentials and training do you have?** Surgeons who are board-certified adhere to a strict code of rules and ethics, including working only in accredited hospitals and facilities, meeting ongoing continuing education requirements, and obeying strict rules about patient ethics.
- **How many procedures like this one have you performed?** Experience counts when choosing your surgeon. Also, look for someone with recent experience—they'll know the current best practices and the most up-to-date options.
- **What are the risks?** Every surgery has some risk. Ask about the risks and side effects, and weigh these against the benefits before making your decision.
- **Where and how will my surgery be performed?** Will surgery be performed in a hospital, office, or ambulatory facility? Is that facility accredited, meaning that it has passed strict guidelines for safety, hygiene, and more? Also, ask how side effects and complications will be handled after your surgery.

Remember that your comfort level is essential. If you don't feel confident that the doctor is the right choice, or if you feel intimidated when you try to ask questions, keep looking. Your confidence with the results of your augmentation depends on it.

Trusted Online Resources about Breast Implants

THE INTERNET IS FULL OF information about breast implants and breast augmentation. But, like any other popular online topic, sorting the trustworthy information from the nonsense can be tough sometimes. We've gathered some of the more trusted resources on the topic into a single list for your consideration.

AmericanBoardCosmeticSurgery.org

The American Board of Cosmetic Surgery is dedicated to helping patients understand the practice of cosmetic surgery. On the website they have information regarding breast augmentation, including pricing data, before and after pictures, and available options. In addition you can find a cosmetic surgeon in your area, who can further help you understand the nature of aesthetic breast surgery and answer all of your questions.

PlasticSurgery.org

The website of the American Society of Plastic Surgeons provides a wealth of information about breast augmentation surgeries. Learn why people choose breast implants, which options are available, what to expect, and how to choose a doctor with whom you feel completely comfortable.

FDA.gov

From blowing the whistle on the unsafe silicone gel implants of the past to approving today's most up-to-date options and tracking patient complaints, the U.S. Food and Drug Administration (FDA) has become one of the most trusted resources on the topic of breast implants. Learn about the differences between various types of approved and cleared implants, review manufacturers' information and websites, find out what symptoms indicate a complication, and track your implants so you'll be the first to know if there's ever a problem.

MedlinePlus.gov

MedlinePlus provides trusted health information to patients and physicians nationwide on a massive array of topics, including an entire series on breast implants, augmentation, and reconstruction after mastectomy. The site also offers links to other trusted resources, including the American Cancer Society.

RealSelf.com

We include RealSelf.com here because it has become one of the Internet's biggest "hubs" for discussion of breast augmentation and revision surgeries. Users have asked nearly every question imaginable, and most have been answered by at least one physician. While this community shouldn't serve as a replacement for talking to your own doctor, it can offer a valuable support group and help you understand what you should expect—and which questions to ask your doctor to ensure your experience is a positive one.

BabyMed.com

This popular site for baby information covers *a lot* more than just breast implants. But included in its informative articles and planners are a wealth of articles about pregnancy and breastfeeding with implants, including what to expect and how to make sure both you and your baby have a comfortable experience. You can also share experiences and gain insight from other new mothers who have implants.

National Center for Biotechnology Information (NCBI)

As part of the National Institutes of Health (NIH), the NCBI offers access to thousands of research articles, books, studies, and reviews on breast implants and augmentation surgeries through the PubMed database. Any interested member of the public can use the search function on the NCBI website to find the most recently published research and scientific information on breast implants.

The NCBI also offers access to partial or full-text scientific articles, books, and journals on its website. For instance, one book available in the collection is Safety of Silicone Breast Implants, published in 1999 by the Committee on the *Safety of Silicone Breast Implants*. Readers can browse the entire book online or download a PDF version of the text to read at their leisure.

Why Do Men Care about Breast Size?

MALE FASCINATION WITH BREAST SIZE is no secret—and it's also no secret that breasts hold more interest for some men than for others. While theories about the reason for this interest have circulated for centuries, two recent studies reveal that the real reasons for men's attention to women's breast sizes may be more complex than we think.

The first study, conducted by psychologists Viren Swami and Martin Tovée, sought to explore the connection between men's access to resources and their preferences for breast sizes. The researchers hypothesized that because the breasts can signal the body's fat reserves, larger breasts may indicate more access to resources—and thus be more desirable to men who felt themselves to be resource scarce.

The researchers recruited 266 men of varying socioeconomic statuses and showed them animations of women who varied only in their breast sizes. The men were asked to rate the characters' physical attractiveness on a five-point scale. The researchers found that, indeed, men of lower socioeconomic status were more likely to find large breasts appealing than men of higher socioeconomic status. A second study performed on men who were just going to a meal versus men who had just finished a meal found that men also like larger breasts when they themselves are hungrier—in other words, when their bodies feel resource scarce.

In a second study, researchers Christopher Burris and Armand Munteanu explored the perceived connection between breast size and ability to bear healthy children. In their study, Burris and Munteanu asked 67 men to rate their desires to become fathers, then to use a computer program to create their ideal female body proportions. Once again, the study found a correlation: the men who indicated a strong desire not to have children preferred smaller breasts, while the men who indicated a strong desire to become fathers preferred larger breasts.

These studies indicate that there are some sound evolutionary reasons that some men pay close attention to breast size, and why others may rate smaller breasts more attractive. Female confidence and comfort may also play a role. Put another way, a woman who feels comfortable and attractive due to her breast size and symmetry may appear more confident and approachable, gaining the attention of potential partners.

Breast Enhancement: Psychological Benefits

FROM A PHYSICAL STANDPOINT, THE benefits of breast enhancement include improving breast symmetry, raising a sagging chest profile, and reconstructing the breasts after surgery or another major life event. But many people don't realize that the mental and emotional health benefits of breast enhancement can greatly outweigh these physical benefits.

Here are just a few of the ways in which a breast enhancement can contribute to psychological health:

1. **Improved Self-Esteem**

Patients who know what to expect from their breast enhancement and work carefully with their surgeon to choose the right size and style of implant for their desired results often report increased self-esteem and self-confidence once they healed from their surgeries. Looking better in your clothes and feeling more comfortable in your body can do much to help you carry yourself more confidently and enjoy life, rather than feeling anxious and insecure.

2. **Reduced Body Dysphoria**

In extreme cases, anxiety over one's looks or body shape isn't mere insecurity—it becomes a psychological condition known as "dysphoria," in which the body feels "wrong" in a way that causes acute mental and emotional distress. Some mastectomy patients, for example, experience dysphoria after one or both breasts are removed, because it feels "wrong" that a part of their body is no longer present. Breast enhancement can work as part of an overall plan to treat and alleviate dysphoria.

3. **Sexual Function**

In most cases, breast enhancement surgery does not reduce a person's enjoyment of sexual or sensual play regarding the breasts—and many people report that they actually enjoy these activities *more* once their breast enhancement has fully healed. While some reports of greater enjoyment appear to be related to physical changes in the nerves of the breasts, others are linked to the mental and emotional benefits of feeling more beautiful, attractive, or desirable.

These mental and emotional health benefits can have positive effects in other areas of one's life as well. For instance, feeling more confident and comfortable in your body may help you focus on your work or find the courage to ask for the raise you deserve, improving your work life as well as your personal self-esteem. To fully reap the benefits of a breast enhancement, it is important to be informed about the options and limitations of the surgery and to work with a doctor you trust.

Dubious "Natural Breast Enlargement" Therapies

TYPE THE WORDS "BREAST ENLARGEMENT" into your favorite search engine, and the results will include thousands or even millions of hits for pills, creams, herbs, exercises, and other recommendations that promise to improve your bustline in a "natural" or even "risk-free" manner. These promises, however, are often overblown—and sometimes dangerous.

Here are some of the most common "natural breast enlargement" therapies offered, as well as their promises and their risks:

1. **Supplements**

Several companies sell "breast enlargement supplements" that claim to offer a natural means to increase breast size. They typically contain a list of herbal ingredients, some of which mimic the way estrogen behaves in the human body. Ingredients that may appear in these supplements include black cohosh root, dong quai (a Chinese herb), fennel, fenugreek, saw palmetto, wild yam, and kava, along with "filler" grains like barley, hops, or oats.

These products are rarely tested for efficacy. In the United States, they often are not tested by the U.S. Food and Drug Administration (FDA). While certain active herbal ingredients can change the body's hormonal levels, they may not result in larger breasts, but may lead to hormonal imbalances, according to the Mayo Clinic.

2. **Creams**

Patients who don't want to take a supplement pill may turn to one of the many "breast enlargement creams" available for sale. Some of these creams contain hormonal additives that operate similarly to the herbs used in "natural" supplement pills, while others include little more than a few oils and vitamins the same ingredients found in any skin lotion.

While the risk of using a cream depends on the ingredients in the cream itself, no breast enlargement cream has been shown to change the size of the breasts. In most cases, those who purchase these creams are simply paying a premium for ordinary lotion.

3. **Exercises**

Exercises generally do not increase the size of the breast itself. However, certain exercises—those that work the pectoral muscles of the chest—can increase the size and firmness of this muscle, which can help the breast tissue stand out. This can give the appearance of a larger breast.

While exercise does not pose the same risks as taking an untested pill or cream, it is important to check with your doctor to make sure you are healthy enough for exercise. It's also important to recognize the limits of what exercising the pectoral muscles can do for your bust size.

Taking Care of Your Breasts

WHETHER OR NOT YOU ARE considering a breast enlargement, it's important to keep breasts healthy. Breast health not only helps you reduce the risk of cancer, it also helps your breasts look their best.

While "quick fix" pills or creams won't do much to improve the look or health of your breasts, there are many steps you can take to ensure that your breasts look great and stay their healthiest throughout your lifespan. Here's a "quick start" guide to doing just that:

1. **Eat well.**

A healthy diet isn't just good for your overall health—it's great for your breasts too. A diet that seeks to balance macronutrient groups (protein, carbs, and fats) and that limits processed sugars, highly processed carbs and polyunsaturated vegetable oils may have cancer-fighting benefits. It also helps maintain your overall body health, of which your breasts are an integral part.

2. Exercise.

The Mayo Clinic recommends that adults get 30 minutes of moderate exercise or 15 minutes of vigorous exercise five days a week. Exercise helps improve blood flow and boosts your body's ability to rid itself of toxins, which improves the health of the breasts and other tissues. A wide range of activities count as moderate exercise, from walking to gardening to impromptu dance parties in your living room.

To give your breasts an added exercise "boost," focus on strength-building exercises that work the shoulders, back, core, and pectoral muscles. This will help your posture and will strengthen the areas around your breasts, both of which will help maintain your bustline.

3. Get some sun—but not too much.

A little sun every day helps your body maintain its stores of vitamin D, which is essential to help fight fatigue, improve mood, and process other vitamins and minerals. If you can't get outdoors, try installing a full-spectrum lightbulb in your office or living room, to mimic the effects of natural sunlight.

While a little sun is essential, too much can be harmful to your breast health. If you're going to be outside for extended periods, don't forget to put on sunblock, cover up, and to drink plenty of water.

Hormonal Influences on Breast Size

AS MANY WOMEN KNOW, THE rhythms of your hormonal cycle or the hormonal changes that come with pregnancy can greatly change the sensitivity, shape, and even the size of your breasts. Hormonal factors do influence breast size, and certain steps can be taken to change your hormonal balance.

Here are some of the more common hormonal factors that influence breast size and what can be done about them:

1. Estrogen

Estrogen plays a significant role in breast growth. However, too much estrogen may result in an imbalance in your overall hormonal profile, which can lead to a number of problematic symptoms. Added estrogen may have certain side effects as well, such as an increased risk of breast cancer or certain reproductive cancers. If you're seeking to include estrogen in your system, the best way to do so is to talk to a doctor who can help you manage any side effects and prepare for the risks.

2. Progesterone

Estrogen and progesterone are "partners" in the menstrual cycle, and both play a role in breast size and sensitivity. While over-the-counter progesterone products are available, they may pose similar risks as estrogen in terms of hormonal imbalance or increased cancer risk.

3. Prolactin

During puberty and pregnancy, the body produces higher amounts of prolactin, which helps develop the mammary glands and increase stores of fat in the breasts. This, in turn, changes the size and shape of the breasts in many people.

4. Growth Hormone

Human growth hormone (HGH) affects the growth of every part of the body, including the breasts. While most people's bodies produce this hormone naturally in childhood, it's important to make sure your HGH levels are appropriate to your body size, type, and age. Merely adding HGH won't target breast growth, and it may have other unwanted side effects.

Genetics play the single biggest role in your breast shape and size, and in how your hormones operate to affect breast shape and size. Your DNA affects everything from the amount of breast tissue you have and its location to your skin quality and the strength of the ligaments and other parts of the breasts.

Tips on Choosing the Right Size Implant

BREAST AUGMENTATION IS A HIGHLY personal decision, and so is the process of choosing the implant size that is best for you.

Many people rate "trying on" implants as the most fun part of preparing for a breast augmentation surgery. Typically, you'll try on various implant sizes at your doctor's office, with the help of staff members who can answer your questions and give you any feedback you request. You may be asked to bring along a few different types of shirts or tops, so you can see how your completed augmentation is likely to look with your wardrobe.

When you look for the right size implant for you, keep these tips in mind:

1. Describe what you want in terms of your body size and shape.

Some people want a "natural" look that is indistinguishable from how your breasts might have grown in on their own; others want their implants to be more noticeable. When describing what you want, don't hesitate to talk about location, height, and shape with reference to your own body.

The one reference point to avoid? Cup sizes. Bra cup sizes are a little different for each manufacturer, so simply saying you want to be a "D cup," for example, may not help be helpful when trying to find the right implant size for you.

2. Give each set of implants several minutes before you decide.

It can be startling at first to see yourself with extra "padding" in your bustline. Instead of altogether rejecting the implant you're trying on, take a few minutes to examine yourself in the mirror. Look at yourself from various angles. Imagine what you will feel like getting up every morning and seeing this difference without clothing. If the change feels "right" to you, you're on the right track. If it feels too large or too small, move on.

3. Take photos.

It's always wise to go home and think about your options before making your final decision. To help you do this, make sure you get front, angle, side, and back photographs of yourself trying on each implant size, in your bra and in one or more tops. This will help you compare and consider at home, and to ask for input from loved ones or close friends if you want it.

Should You Wait until after Having Children?

PREGNANCY AND BREASTFEEDING OFTEN CHANGE the size, shape, and sensitivity of breasts, as anyone who has ever been pregnant or breastfed her child knows. As a result, it's important to consider whether or not to wait until you've added all the children you wish to your family before you have breast augmentation surgery.

Here are a few key points to consider when deciding when to plan your breast augmentation:

Breast implants do not affect fertility. According to the U.S. Food and Drug Administration (FDA) and to countless people who have had babies after a breast augmentation, breast implants do not make it harder to conceive or increase your risk of miscarriage.

Having breast implants will not affect your baby's health. Multiple studies, following thousands of mothers and infants, have discovered no link between breast implants and birth defects or health problems in babies—even babies who were breastfed by mothers with implants. These studies have been conducted on both silicone and saline implants with the same results.

However, it is also important to consider that:

Pregnancy may change your breasts—and the results of your surgery. Your age when you get pregnant, the age and type of your implants, the characteristics of your breast tissue, and how your breast tissue changes during pregnancy might affect your breast size, shape, or profile with implants, just as it would without implants. Or it may not. Talk to other women in your family to find out how pregnancy affected their breasts, as genetics plays a key role in these results.

Breastfeeding may be affected by implants—or it may not. Studies indicate that most women who have breast implants can breastfeed their babies, and that the breastfeeding does not negatively affect either the baby or the breast augmentation. Since implants are placed below the breast tissue and milk ducts, the implant should not affect your ability to produce milk or for your baby to access it.

However, not all women can breastfeed naturally, whether or not they have implants. While you can't always predict whether or not you'll be able to breastfeed, you can ask other women in your family to share their experiences, and talk to your doctors, so you have a better idea what to expect.

Ten Key Things to Consider before Having Surgery

OUR SERIES ON BREAST AUGMENTATION covered a wide range of topics, from the details of the procedure itself to how to decide whether a breast augmentation is right for you. It's a lot of information to digest. Here are the top ten takeaways to consider before your breast augmentation surgery:

1. Do it for you.

Increased self-confidence, comfort in your body, and contentment with yourself are great reasons to have a breast augmentation. The not-so-great reasons? Anything that involves impressing—or ending the pressure from—someone else.

2. Get expert advice (and a little help from your friends).

Make sure your information about incisions, implant placement, implant types, and surgical care are coming from sources with experience performing breast augmentation surgeries. But don't hesitate to ask your friends for some advice on sizes, scheduling, or self-care.

3. Understand the risks and the benefits.

Like all surgeries, breast augmentation comes with certain risks. Make sure you know what these are, and that you understand the benefits to expect, so you're fully prepared to make smart choices about your health.

4. Prepare to handle the costs.

Unfortunately, many insurance companies don't cover breast augmentation surgery (or potential complications). Get quotes and compare prices, so you can budget effectively. The last thing you need is to stress about the bill!

5. Consider all your options.

Silicone, saline, or gel implants? Under the muscle or over it? Incision below the breast, or somewhere else? Get the facts, so you can choose the best options for the results you want.

6. Don't DIY.

"Natural" breast enhancement creams, pills, or other gadgets aren't harmless—and they almost never provide the results you want. Work with a professional surgeon instead.

7. Play dress-up.

Take all the time you need to try on implant sizes, compare photos, and choose the size and shape that are going to make you feel most comfortable with your body.

8. Prepare for a successful surgery.

Avoid smoking, get plenty of rest, and pay careful attention to instructions on when to stop eating or drinking, so your surgery can avoid unnecessary complications and you can heal more quickly.

9. Take care of yourself.

Schedule downtime after surgery to rest and relax. The better you rest, the more quickly and fully your body can heal—and the sooner you can fully enjoy the results of your surgery.

10. Choose a doctor you trust.

It's wise to talk to several surgeons before you choose the one you'll want to perform the surgery. We're ready to answer your questions and help you make an informed choice at any time. Just give our office a call.

Before and After

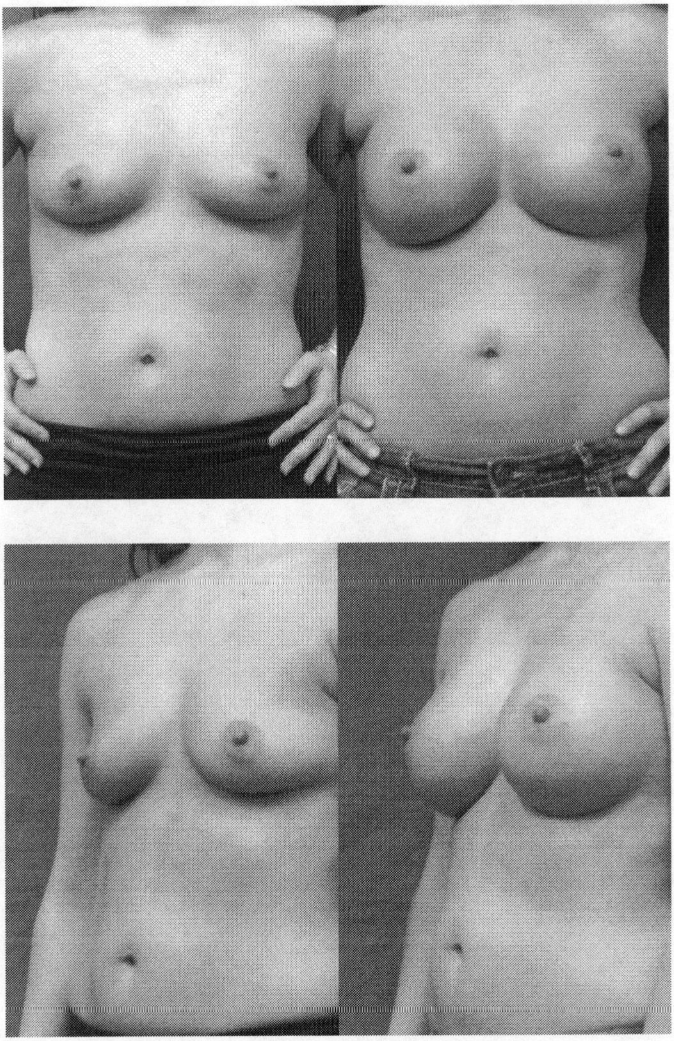

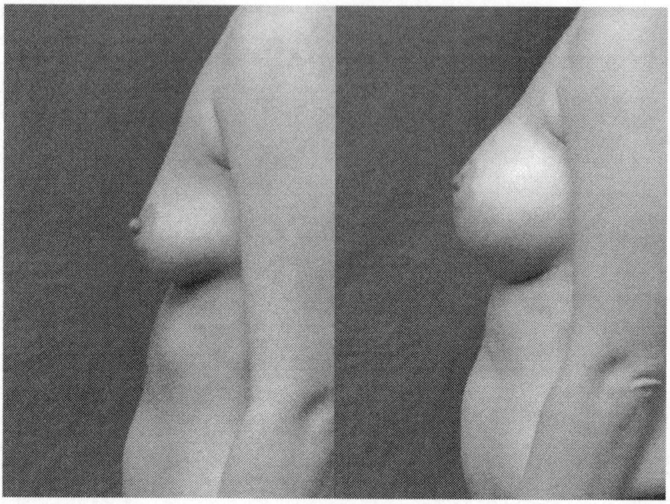

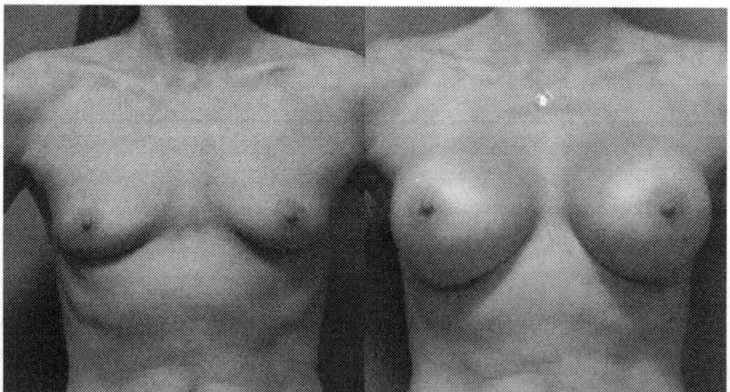

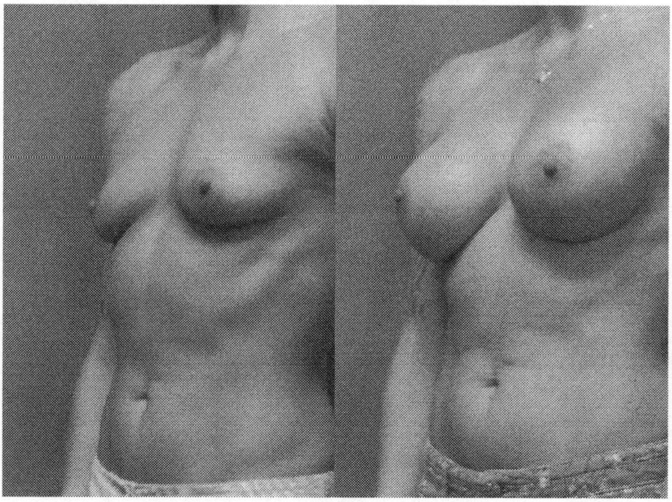

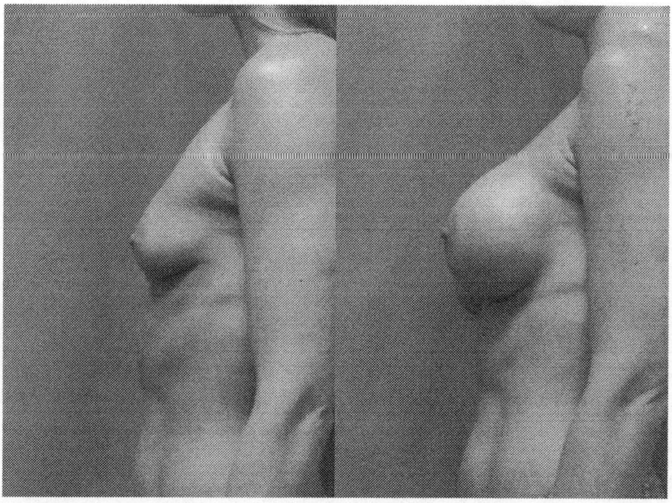

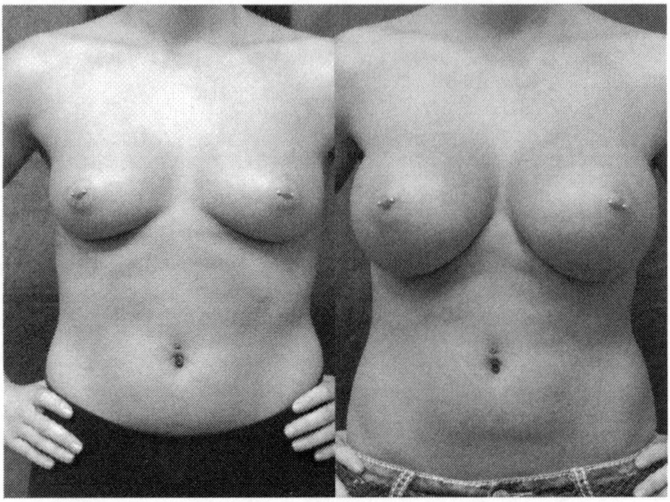

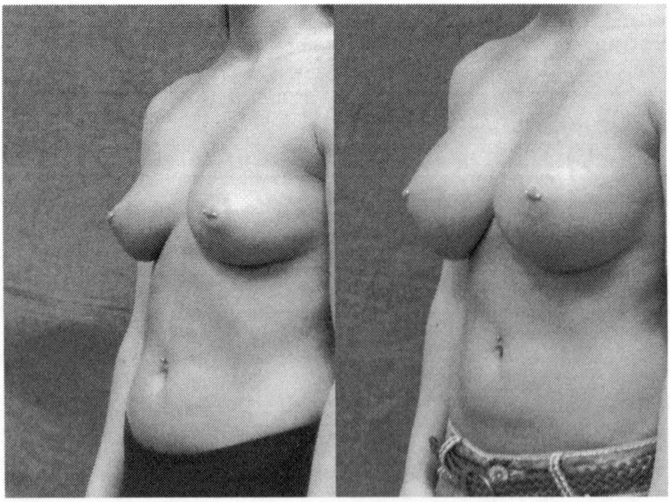

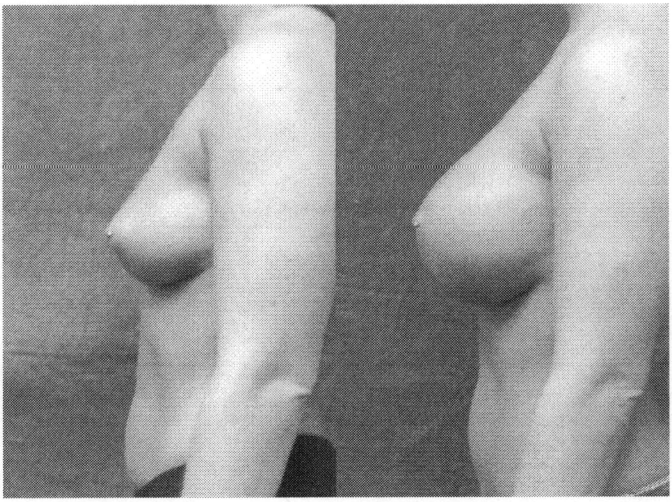

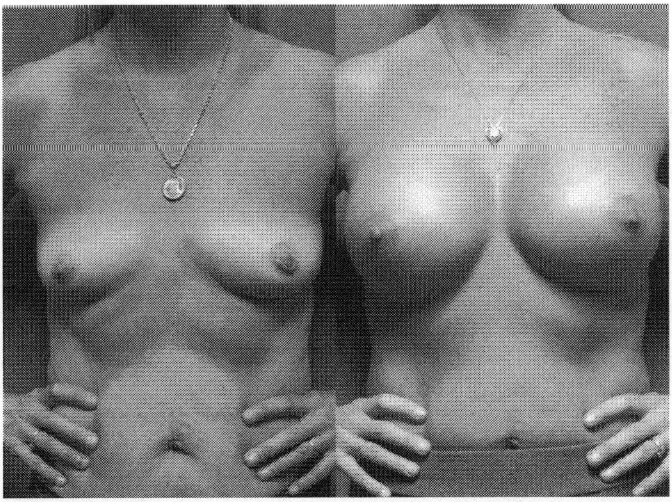

Conclusion

WE'VE GONE ON A LONG journey together—this wasn't called the *Big* Book of Boobs for no reason—and hopefully you now have a much deeper insight into what actually happens during this surgery and what you can expect.

In addition to exploring the nuts and bolts of the process, we shared some historical and cultural perspective, so you can understand the procedure in context.

While we made an effort to cover as many commonly asked questions as we could, it's possible—likely, even—that you have specific concerns about your options, constraints, time frame, or unique medical situation. Our team is standing by to help. Please call the office today at (216) 264-8100 to speak with us and get smart advice about your next steps.

Thanks again for taking the time to read this book, and good luck!

About Our Practice

DR. MATT GOLDSCHMIDT AT THE Cosmetic Surgery Center offers all of the most common and gratifying cosmetic surgery procedures. Some of the procedures he performs include breast augmentation, liposuction, facelift, breast lift, tummy tuck, eyelid surgery, facial fillers, and Botox. He is passionate about cosmetic surgery and has performed thousands of surgeries over his career. He has put together a team of care providers in Cleveland, Ohio, who are dedicated to helping you achieve the best results possible. He is an expert in the field of cosmetic surgery. He has published papers in this field, has given many lectures, and serves as an examiner for the American Board of Cosmetic Surgery.

In addition, he is committed to helping less fortunate individuals and families through his philanthropic endeavors. You will be amazed at how well you will be cared for when you come to The Cosmetic Surgery Center in Cleveland, Ohio.

The office is conveniently located off of I-77 and I-480 in the Crown Centre Building in Independence, Ohio. This location makes it easy for patients coming from Western Pennsylvania, Youngstown, Akron, Canton, Dayton, and Toledo.

Disclaimer

Disclaimer for *The Big Book of Boobs*:

You understand that this book is not intended as a substitution for a consultation with a breast implant surgeon, and it is not medical advice.

Requesting this book or viewing the information in it does not create a doctor-patient relationship with Dr. Matt Goldschmidt or The Cosmetic Surgery Center. To obtain medical advice, please engage the services of The Cosmetic Surgery Center or another qualified medical practice of your choice. To discuss engaging The Cosmetic Surgery Center to help you with your medical needs, please contact the practice.

DR. MATT GOLDSCHMIDT AND THE COSMETIC SURGERY CENTER ARE PROVIDING *THE BIG BOOK OF BOOBS* (HEREAFTER REFERRED TO AS "BOOK") AND ITS CONTENTS ON AN "AS IS" BASIS AND MAKES NO REPRESENTATIONS OR WARRANTIES OF ANY KIND WITH RESPECT TO THIS BOOK OR ITS CONTENTS. DR. MATT GOLDSCHMIDT AND THE COSMETIC SURGERY CENTER DISCLAIM ALL SUCH REPRESENTATIONS AND WARRANTIES, INCLUDING, FOR EXAMPLE, WARRANTIES OF MERCHANTABILITY AND FITNESS FOR A PARTICULAR PURPOSE. IN ADDITION, DR. MATT GOLDSCHMIDT AND THE COSMETIC SURGERY CENTER DO NOT REPRESENT OR WARRANT THAT THE

INFORMATION ACCESSIBLE VIA THIS BOOK IS ACCURATE, COMPLETE, OR CURRENT.

The book is provided for informational purposes only, and relevant medical knowledge frequently changes. Except as specifically stated in this book, neither Dr. Matt Goldschmidt nor The Cosmetic Surgery Center nor any authors, contributors, or other representatives will be liable for damages arising out of or in connection with the use of this book. This is a comprehensive limitation of liability that applies to all damages of any kind, including (without limitation) compensatory; direct, indirect, or consequential damages; loss of data, income or profit; loss of or damage to property, and claims of third parties and punitive damages.

Made in the USA
Monee, IL
08 November 2026

67380763R00060